CHRONIC RHEUMATISM

by

Dr. Fortier-Bernoville

&

Dr. L. A. Rousseau

(Translated from the Original French)

by

Dr. Rajkumar Mukerji

M.A., L.H.M.S.

B. Jain Publishers Pvt. Ltd.

NEW DELHI-110055

Reprint 1987

Price : Rs. 3.00

Publishers :   B. Jain Publishers Pvt. Ltd.
1921, Chuna Mandi, Street 10th,
NEW DELHI-110055 (INDIA)

Printed in   : J. J. Offset Printers
India by   Pharganj, New Delhi-110055

PREFACE

The articles included in this little book are translations from articles originally published in the French language in the journal l' Homoeopathie Moderne.

The first article is a translation of the article "Traitement homoeopathique du Rhumatisme chronique", by Dr. Fortier-Bernoville published in l' Homoeopathie Moderne No. 8, 15th April, 1935 and the article on "Sciatica" is a translation of the article "Sciatique" by Dr. L.A. Rousseau published in the same journal No. 5, 1st March, 1935. The article "acute articular rheumatism" is also by Dr. Fortier-Bernoville published in the same journal.

For the explanation of the words "drainage" the readers are referred to my translation *What we must not do in Homoeopathy*, published by Jain Publishers of New Delhi.

I hope this little book will be useful to homoeopathic practitioners in their daily practice.

Chandarnagor
September 1975.

—Raj Kumar Mukerji

PREFACE

The articles included in this little book are translations from articles originally published in the French language in the journal l' Homoeopathie Moderne.

The first article is a translation of the article "Traitement homoeopathique du Rhumatisme chronique", by Dr. Fortier-Bernoville published in l' Homoeopathie Moderne No. 8, 15th April, 1935 and the article on "Sciatica" is a translation of the article "Sciatique" by Dr. I.A. Rousseau published in the same journal No. 5, 1st March, 1935. The article "acute articular rheumatism" is also by Dr. Fortier-Bernoville published in the same journal.

For the explanation of the words "drainage", the readers are referred to my translation What we must not do in Homoeopathy, published by Jain Publishers of New Delhi.

I hope this little book will be useful to homoeopathic practitioners in their daily practice.

—Raj Kumar Mukerji

Chandarnagor
September 1975.

Chronic Rheumatism

Gentlemen

When you asked me the other day to prepare this subject of therapeutics, I accepted it without taking into account the difficulties to overcome and I did not think that an introduction on this subject will be such a delicate problem. I thought that I was competent to answer the question of homoeopathic treatment of chronic rheumatism. Every week I treat a number of rheumatic patients. I treat them with or without success according to the cases ; however, I generally get good results, but also like any other doctor, there are some failures, which humiliate me and the humiliation is a good quality of a doctor, which checks the momentary exaggerated or dangerous enthusiasm.

Nevertheless, I thought that it was easy to classify and hierarchise the remedies. When I wanted to put it down on paper, I was at first surprised to see the difficulty to solve the problem and I asked myself, if I will have to write a complete book in order to solve the problem because if we want to study fully the medicines of Chronic Rheumatism, we will not be able to finish it within this short space. It is a very wide field. On the one hand the remedies proposed by different doctors are numerous and on the other hand the opinions are very different and controversial on their values. It is difficult to put an order in them. Some homoeopathic medicines are very active, the others have questionable value. But the question of doses for many remedies has not yet been solved and above all etiology and pathology of the different forms of chronic rheumatism are hardly yet described, not only in Allopathy but also in Homoeopathy.

It is true that in homoeopathy we can cure some rheumatic patients whose conditions discouraged the Officials ; it is also certain and we must admit our failures, and that sometimes we do not get any result.

It is therefore necessary to try to understand what is chronic rheumatism and how we can treat it. Homoeopathy is a philosophy. Its principal quality is to give to the practitioner "a turn of mind" which is very different to that of the doctors of the other School. We have, as diciples of Hahnemann, some ideas that are as much the "supported" as those of biologists, but these ideas are the keys by their general character of fecundity and of clearness, and schematic simplicity. We will have to give to the intuitive genius of Hahnemann some experimental basis as regards Psora, Sycosis etc.

Those who will follow us will perhaps teach to the students who have come to Homoeopathy a scheme probably very different to that which we are giving here and which is valuable only for the present.

Etiology, Ground Treatment and Nosodes

As regards etiology there are some nosodes which correspond to the real factors of rheumatism. The most important is the Psora of Hahnemann, which we see appear again and again. This Psora is an important hereditary taint more or less augmented by acquired toxins which follow us and which cause rheumatism in predisposed persons. In an etiological way, all diluted *Tuberculins* will therefore be used in persons suffering from rheumatism.

I am inclined to believe that our friend **Dr.** Martiny will just now give us some notions about pathogenesis and etiology of this disease in the light of the recent works on biology and I hope that you will not hesitate to take side with his opinion.

The question of *Tuberculins* play an important part in chronic rheumatism as ground remedies. *Medorrhinum*, the nosode of gonorrhoea and *Syphilinum* are less important of these two factors the gonorrhoeal poison is of the second importance and syphilis the third in importance. But before speaking of these two entities let me speak of Psora at first.

The Psora may be neutralised by diluted *Tuberculins* which you will give to the patient after having drained him well, after having prescribed the necessary ground remedies and the functional remedies.

By the side of this classical Psora, which can be individualised by the different *Tuberculins* we may also fight against this type of affection by *nosodes* of *Bach*, a new product prepared out of the culture of microbes of intestinal origin prepared by Bach, an Englishman.

The toxin remedies of *Cahis* of which we have said while speaking about acute rheumatism are equally interesting. Cahis usually divided the persons suffering from rheumatism into two groups ; those who have chronic suppurations of the throat, of gums and those who do not suffer from them. It is necessary we should pay homage to the author who have had the idea before the American authors who have shown the importance of suppuration, chronic or latent of the cavum, dental infections and infections of tonsils that are capable to produce all sorts of diseases.

When he treats a patient who has no trouble of teeth or gums, he gives *Rheumatoxin, i.e..* a remedy prepared with a drop of blood of the patient suffering from acute rheumatism.   When on the contrary the patient has unhealthy teeth, specially pyorrhoea he gives *Pyorrhin.* The dilutions are 18th to 5000.

You can also act in this manner by *Oscillococcin* of J. Roy or by an isopathy prepared from the urine of the patient.

I was saying just now that Psora, to which correspond therapeutically different *Tuberculins* that play the most important part as regards etiology of chronic rheumatism for homoeopaths.   But very often gonococcus is associated with this miasm.   Then you have a person who was a *tuberculinic* while a child or an adolescent becuase he was in a very unhealthy situation or he inherited tubercular taints from his parents.   He is therefore a typical psoric subject of Hahnemann, because he contracts for example gonorrhoea at the age of 18 to 20 and after sometime even if he does suffer from acute rheumatism, he may at first have symptoms of sub-acute rheumatism, then chronic rheumatism in which the two etiologies, the tuberculinic toxin and gonorrhoea toxin are intricated.

Also in patients in whom we have amelioration of rheumatism by the ground remedies and 'the drainage remedies, we have incorporated in their treatment high dilutions of *Tuberculin* on the one hand and *Medorrhinum* on the other hand, and we get clearly superior results.

I open here a parenthesis as regards this touchstone treatment. Perhaps I am wrong to use this term because in homoeopathy as well as in allopathy we have the tendency to think that every time we use a remedy called specific and when the remedy acts, it follows that the etiology of which we are thinking is really the cause. But this is not true. It is possible that *Medorrhinum* has acted homoeopathically in persons whose toxins are due to *diplococcus* or *gonococcus*, but not identifiable with the latter. Cahis has brought a revolution as regards that question in homoeopathy, using for example *Meningococcin* in the place of *Medorrhinum*. By giving some nosodes without taking into account of the specificity and only according to the similarity or characteristics, one can get also some results if these nosodes are used according to the law of similars.

In the third place, syphilis may play an important part in some rheumatic patients, specially in persons who have articular or bone deformations. But this factor seems secondary and distant in relation to gonococcic or tuberculinic toxins.

Dr. Martiny is now going to give us some ideas on the biology of this question.

Dr. Martiny—My friend Fortier-Bernoville has taken me quite unprepared. I have not studied the question of chronic rheumatism before entering this hall. It is certain that it is the question of real life and to give a therapeutics of chronic rheumatism is already very difficult and a biological explanation is much more delicate.

In the last congress on rheumatism of which the presidents were M. BesaCon and Mr. Mathieu Pierre Weil, very interesting controversies took place. Every one had his classification, his conception. There was no agreement and one had the impression that he knew more while entering than while coming out of the congress. The few clear ideas that one could have about clinical and therapeutic spheres and also thought rarely on biological sphere, disappeared at the end of a moment.

From the practical point of view however, in the chaos, what surprised me was the fact that one was wrong to call under the name of chronic rheumatism some diseases that have no relations amongst themselves.

As for example if an old man has arthritis of his hips it is called chronic rheumatism. It has however, no relation with diffused neuralgia from which a young man may suffer, neither with deforming rheumatism.

If one wishes to simplify the problem, it would be necessary to precise the known symptoms of chronic rheumatism. It is necessary to differentiate the chronic rheumatism from acute rheumatism which has become chronic *i.e.* to say from all subacute rheumatism (the subject suffering from subacute rheumatism becomes later on patients of articular rheumatism or rheumatism of articulations). An infectious rheumatism like that of gonorrhoeal rheumatism should be considered separately. The name rheumatism should be reserved only for rheumatism of which the cause is unknown.

If one looks at the chart of Dr. Fortier Bernoville, one will find two spheres of the question, the superior sphere and the etiological sphere. The causes appear to be *tuberculosis syphilis dental alveolar pyorrhoea*. The lower sphere is symptomatic. There one will find the functional remedies, organotherapy and classical homoeopathy. It is the sphere of the ground, of the manifestations of the disease. One starts from the ground to arrive at the causes.

Probing into the deep causes we find the organs which are more involved than the others. One can also describe thyroidean rheumatism, the gland being very often involved. The liver troubles are important. We may also say that troubles of assimilation are among the important causes. As regards the kidneys, I think that, the affections are not of the first order like the liver troubles. The rheumatism due to the troubles of the pituitary gland is classical. The patient suffers from pains of all the limbs. Let us not forget also the importance of the parathyroid.

I have left aside the chemical causes, the metabolism of *Calcium*, of *Potassium*, of *Alcalosis*. The biology of rheumatism is perhaps much more subtle. It is certain, that rheumatism has endocrinal troubles, consequently, troubles of biological resonances. It is interesting to build the bridge between these troubles and those of vitaminosis. If this question is enlarged we will find more and more the importance of food which will justify to a certain point the ideas of *Carton* and *Bircher*.

We must keep in mind as etiology the idea of sedentarism. It is good to speak about microbes, but the manner in which we live is also important.

Let us keep in mind the relation between Psora and Tuberculosis. The tuberculous rheumatism of *Poncet* is becoming more and more important. From the humoral point of view the rheumatism is more related to tuberculosis. *Vernes resorsin* reaction has a great importance in the appreciation of chronic tuberculous and rheumatic states, taking into account the series of acute manifestations. What brings the researches to think tuberculosis as the principal cause of rheumatism is that, studying rheumatism humorally, one has discovered sensibilising causes which are related to the sensitiveness to tuberculosis. The tuberculous toxin is very special ; it is allergising *i.e.* secondary. The *tuberculin* injected in a healthy person does not produce any effect. But it is a secondary toxin, very rich in proteins which helps to relate tuberculous diseases to serum diseases.

It is curious to note that tuberculous rheumatism is very rare in persons suffering from tuberculosis in evolution, and it appears in persons who had tuberculosis, but does not suffer from it any more, which means that arthritism fights tuberculosis.

Today we may ask if it is not simply a manifestation of rarefication of *tuberculin* in the humors. When the person secretes through an opening high doses of tuberculin in his humors, it creates a desensibilisation according to a natural technique of Bisredka type.

When on the contrary, the *tuberculin* is rarified, and it is really what happens when the tuberculous patients are cured, it is at that moment when that infinitesimal tuberculin becomes sensibilising. The diluted antigen becomes antebody. The rheumatic phenomena may be produced by themechanism of antebody-antigen reaction. Besides homoeopathic *tuberculins* act admirably in tuberculosis.

The idea of the influence of *tuberculin* chronic on rheumatism is therefore important. Very important is also the influence of dental pyorrhoea. But this type of rheumatism is very different and may be more easily corrected when one thinks of it. With this rheumatism may be compared all the rheumatisms resulting out of microbian digestive troubles (*streptococcus and enterococcus*).

The gonococcic toxin like that of syphilitic toxin, like all other secondary toxins having tendency to allergic condition, cause predisposition to rheumatism.

In summary we may say that a rheumatic subject is by his constitution an endocrinian and weakly intoxinated by the toxins that he carries within him. He is a sensitive person and his sensitiveness may cause rheumatic affections.

In chronic rheumatism there is a tendency to *alcalosis*. Now Dr. Fortier-Bernoville will resume his lecture.

HYDROMINERAL AND PHYSIOTHERAPIC CURE

Before proceeding further let me speak a few words about other methods that are taken recourse to for the treatment of rheumatism. We may also use them, that does not mean a treason to our master Hahneman. We must send our patients to mineral water springs because they are beneficial and they enter into the field of Homoeopathic philosophy.

It is interesting to classify these mineral waters. I believe that the best classification will be Sulphur springs and springs of radio-active waters.

From the clinical point of view what is interesting is to find out up to what point the mineral water treatment is beneficial for a patient who is being treated by Homoeopathy. Some persons for example who have got no amelioration during a season in Dax (a Sulphur spring station) ; who were then treated homoeopathically and who have retired to that station, have obtained clear amelioration thanks to the homoeopathic treatment which preceded his stay....

All mineral water stations may be beneficial but they give good effects only after a homoeopathic treatment on condition that physiotherapic treatment has also been made.

Finally it must be said that rheumatism may be cured if the patient wants to be cured. This is the true criterium, he will be cured of chronic rheumatism. The patient who does not wish to remain in his bed year in and year out, is ameliorated because he fights against ankylosis. Inversely he who is very idle becomes ankylosed more and more. The factor "Patient" is very important.

REMEDIES OF TEMPERAMENTS

After having made a review of the nosodes and etiological treatment we are now going to study the homoeopathic remedies. We will rather give the lists of remedies than their indications of all their symptoms ; not only that it seems to me more rational but because if I speak in detail about all the remedies that may be used, it will become very long.

We have placed the ground remedies or remedies of temperaments on our chart in the following manner : In the middle *Natrum sulphuricum* and near it *Thuja* and *Lycopodium*, then on the right side *Causticum, Silicea, Pulsatilla, Cimicifuga.* On the left *Sulphur* and *Calcarea carbonica* (*Phosphorus, Aurum matallicum, Naturum muriaticum* and *Petroleum* may also be considered as ground remedies).

We have underlined three times *Natrum sulphuricum* because it merits to be placed in the first rank in chronic hydrogenoid rheumatism. This remedy has a very deep action. It is *Thuja* that will act deeply. It develops towards chronicity with very marked deficiency of liver and kidneys. We have no need to give here a complete picture of hydrogenoid subject. We must base ourselves on the general etiology. We must not have the idea that this remedy is used in persons living near a lake or in damp places. It is a remedy of persons living in unsalubrious humid places with less ventilation and sun. We must also keep in mind that the hydrogenoid condition may not only exist in fat persons but also in lean persons having aggravation before a storm.

It is therefore necessary to think first of all about *Natrum sulphuricum.* In its etiology very often *Psora* and *Gonococcus* are found ; the latter frequently plays a part in the antecedents of subjects of the type of *Natrum sulphuricum.*

In this connection I cite here the case of one of my war friends who, in 1947, had gonorrhoea with rheumatism for which he was to be confined for three years. He was treated and cured. He was married and after three years, he began to have rheumatism. I was at that time doing my studies. I tried to treat him, knowing that he had gonorrhoea. The last fact was investigated. Nothing was found. Anti-gonorrheal vaccins caused a terrible aggravation. He left Paris for Lille (where the climate is more cold). Aggravation manifested. Faculty of Lille obtained no result. He could no more walk. He came back to Paris. I tried *Thuja*, *Causticum* and all other remedies with little effect because then I did not know Homoeopathy well. I obtained no result. One day *Natrum sulphuricum* gave fantastic results. But the barrage was not lifted. I tried *Medorrhinum* I failed. Then I gave *T. R.* and I obtained staggering amelioration. He was completely impotent, and could finally walk like any other person at the end of 18 months. We have then re-examined his urethra but nothing was found but since two years he has given gonorrhoea to his wife. Gonococcus was there undetected.

Natrum sulphuricum is therefore an excellent remedy.

Thuja—It has almost the same symptoms as that of *Natrum sulphuricum*. Hydrogenoid constitution and sycosis. But *Thuja* has sometimes less deep action than *Natrum sulphuricum*. The liver is less deficient. It is kidneys that are mainly affected. The patient is aggravated by vaccinations. He had the famous bluish white lower lip.

Causticum—It is also a hydrogenoid of a special character. It has the inverse modality of *Natrum sulphuricum* and *Thuja*. It is hydrogenoid from certain points of view but it is aggravated in dry and fine weather and ameliorated during rain and humidity. But this inverse modality will not last long. Very often the subject of *Causticum* will become a *Rhus Tox*. He will have ankylosis. *Natrum sulphuricum* and *Thuja* have often deforming rheumatism with swelling of articulations. *Causticum* has less swelling of articulations but the patient of *Causticum* will suffer from osteocartilagenous or osteo-muscular rheumatism with muscular paresis and pains irradiating to the right knee. He has pains in hips, aggravated by cough.

Lycopodium goes towards rheumatism because of its insufficient liver and because it does not disintegrate well its ailimentary alcaloids. His rheumatism is ameliorated by the salts of *Lithium*. We will see that salts of *Lithium, Benzioc Acid, Sarsaparilla* and other remedies of the same family are very important complementaries of *Lycopodium* which act in the same sense. Symptoms : Diminution of urea in the urine. Sometimes slight increase of urea in the urine ; less cholestorinemia.

Sulphur is a psoric who has periodic rheumatism alternating with skin troubles, with eczema or digestive troubles. The rheumatic troubles and cutaneous troubles alternate or coexist. The subject has utricaria, furoncles, enterocolitis and diarrhoea. In these cases his rheumatism is ameliorated by sudden stoppage of the diarrhoea.

Calcarea carbonica corresponds to hereditary psora. The subject has articular rheumatism in relation with endocrincial troubles, specially troubles of thyroid and thymus.

Silicea has deforming rheumatism with ankylosis, but has less swelling. It is the inverse of the hydrogenoids, specially of *Natrum sulphuricum* and *Thuja*. Deformations of bones, or in some cases osteo-carti'agineous rheumatism. These are then persons whose swelling of articulations is caused more at the expense of the hard tissues than the soft tissues, of articular tissues properly called. It then affects less peri-articular tissues. There are exceptions because *Silicea* acts on all conjunctive tissues.

Pulsatilla —The subject of *Pulsatilla* has rheumatism as a result of circulatory troubles, specially as a result of venous and capillary congestion. Rheumatism in young persons, more are less tuberculous or tuberculinic. Rheumatism which will have evolution towards *Silicea*. In *Pulsatilla* there is before all an important phenomenon : *erratic pains*. It is a remedy of erratic pains. On the contrary *Natrum sulphuricum*, *Thuja* and *Silicea* have fixed pains.

Cimicifuga (*Actea racemosa*) — Really speaking it is not a remedy of chronic rheumatism. It is rather a remedy of spasms of muscular rheumatism, with jerkings, contractions and cramps. Does *parathyroid* plays a part in *Cimicifuga* ? This question is not yet very clearly explained.

You see then the outline of our homoeopathic treatment of chronic rheumatism by the constitutional remedies. Before passing to the functional remedies we are going to complete the question of the treatment of chronic rheumatism in three or four short chapters.

BIOCHEMIC REMEDIES, ORGANOTHERAPY, DRAINAGE AND LOCAL TREATMENT

Does there exist a class of Homoeopathic remedies which may be called biochemic ? There is such a class. They are less known but they are interesting in the treatment of chronic rheumatism. We know already some biochemic remedies according to the diathesis : *Uric acid, Phosphoric acid, Oxalic acid* corresponding to the three lithiases. You may use these remedies when you have analysed the blood and urine.

Besides these three remedies you must not forget *Nitro muriatic acid*. It is interesting in oxaluria. *Urtica urens, Solidago, Thlaspi*, are plants and may be used as biochemic remedies. We may very often use *Uva ursi* as a drainage remedy.

As I have said above, the question about biochemic remedies is still less known. The question was studied by the Germans in a journal published by a German pharmacy. But the solution is not up to the mark. It is also doubtful whether this question will be ever fully solved. But it is seducing to think that in homoeopathy we have some remedies for which no one can blame us because these remedies have pure laboratory data. Really speaking, Hahnemann was much more wise than most of his successors. He has indicated to us that in order to individualise a patient, it is necessary to do so by his characteristics, by his suggestive symptoms and that often, what we find by the examination of kidneys or analysis of blood. These are the points of arrival and not the points of departure ; points of arrival in relation to extremely different states. We find cholesteronemia or uremia in all sorts of different states. Persons having different temperaments arrive at the same point.

Let us now speak about *organotherapy*. Let our friend Barishac give us some indications on this point.

Dr. Barishac—Classically, the *Thyroid* is regularly used not in the habitual doses which are often ponderable but in infinitesimal doses (200 or 1000). *Parathyroid* and *Pituitary* are often used in deforming rheumatism. For other types of rheumatism they are not so useful.

Dr. Fortier-Bernoville—I must speak at first about general drainage before passing to functional remedies. Besides Homoeopathic drainage which is done on the different spheres, you may also drain the high dilutions. According to the ideas of Dr. Nebel, the drainage done on all possible spheres, the decoctions (*Sarsaparilla, Uva ursi* and still others) may give excellent results. You must remember that many patients were treated and cured thus by Pierre Benoit.

The drainage is then an important question in the treatment of chronic rheumatism. The chronic rheumatism is one of those questions in which Homoeopathy hesitates, does not give much results or acts very slowly. In the latter case the drainage and canalisation are extremely important.

Finally we must not forget that the local treatment in chronic rheumatism is also necessary. The local treatment is rational when you have the troubles of the local tropism such that there exists an antagonism between the local interest of the subject and the general interest of the organism in cause. You may advise local bath to the patient, to apply pommades prepared with the indicated homoeopathic remedies (*Rhus tox* for example); some baths with tincture of *Thuja, Bryonia or Pine oil*, remedies that are more or less empirical, but they act well very often. The same remedies may be used externally.

FUNCTIONAL REMEDIES OR REMEDIES PROPERLY CALLED HOMOEOPATHIC

Let us now speak about functional remedies which are legion. They are numerous because the question of chronic rheumatism has not yet been properly solved. Often we have failures. Gradually as we arrive at a good knowledge about a question and get good results, we make a selection of remedies (As for example we have simplified the treatment of diphtheria in 50 years).

It is impossible to keep in mind all the remedies used in the treatment of chronic rheumatism. Each among us does not use more than 25 to 30 medicines while nearly 150 medicines are indicated in chronic rheumatism. It is often said that one does not cure a patient because one has not used the best remedy. However we must try to find out the good remedy.

Before enumerating the remedies and classifying them in groups, I must insist on a special point. The *localisation.*

The young homoeopath who takes a repertory finds it ridiculous to learn that question when he finds that a remedy is given for the wrist, another for the second phalange of the index of the right arm, another for left knee etc.... For a long time, I also believed that it is stupid to classify the remedies according to the localisations. But such a reasoning is ridiculous because the remedies act according to the local tropism ; there are some affinities in relation to the tissue which we cannot yet explain. It is always Dr. Nebel and his successors who have put the question. It may seem absurd to localise too much. It is homoeopaths who should try in the future to understand well the importance of localisations. In any case we must remember that some remedies have local affinities. It is a very interesting and important question, unfortunately very difficult to answer.

Here is how we have classified the functional and organic remedies of chronic rheumatism.

Let us take up *Calcarea carbonica* with its troubles of metabolism of *Calcium*. By its side we may place *Calcarea Phosphorica* and *Calcarea Fluorica*. The latter acts well in the 3x when you have cartilagineous as well as bone and muscular pains, in persons whose articulations are deformed, whose ligaments become ossified. He begins as for example with a rheumatism of the spinal chord which becomes later on hypertrophysing osteitis. You will often find syphilis in the heredity. *Calcarea carbonica* may be given to big, fat, soft, chilly, hesitating and indolent persons who think that they will never be cured.

Sulphur has digestive and hepatic troubles when he has rheumatism. The very moment he begins to have rheumatism he will require other remedies.

The subject for example has periodic diarrhoeas alternating with rheumatism. You can give him *Dulcamara*. He may have enterocolitis with swelling of the abdomen, false membranes in the stools, aggravation by sweets. He may have arterial hypertension, buzzing in the ears, congestive troubles. He is often a great eater who is never satisfied. He feels weak when he is hungry, feels better after eating. He may have cutaneous troubles in relation with his digestive troubles.

Antimonium crudum is related to *Sulpher*. He is rheumatic, having always a white coated tongue with distended intestines, who feels better after a laxative or if a good intestinal drainage is effected.

Nux vomica may also be used as a complementary to *Sulphur*. By the side of these satellite remedies of *Sulphur* in chronic rheumatism we have an other group that acts on acute articular rheumatism. The best remedies are *Ferrum phosphoricum, Bryonia, Rhus tox. Apis, Pulsatilla*. These remedies will be useful in persons who suffer from rheumatism with occasional and periodic acute or sub-acute inflammation. Suddenly the joints are attacked. It is a form of gouty rheumatism.

Ferrum phosphoricum and *Aconite* have intense pain, dry heat, joints painful to touch, with possible fever but not yet any swelling. *Aconite* has aggravation in dry cold. The subject then passes to the stage of *Bryonia* : amelioration by rest, aggravated by movement pricking pains, painful joints, clear intra-articular rheumatism, often fixed. From *Bryonia* the evolution is towards *Rhus tox* and *Apis*. Both are complementary to *Bryonia* but incompatible. These are two horses of the same harness but they go different directions. *Rhus tox* has the modalities inverse to that of *Bryonia* and we then enter into the group of hydrogenoid remedies which we will soon see. From *Bryonia* the patient goes to *Apis*. The subject will have then all the symptoms of *Apis* ; pale, rosy swellings, pains, redness, but the swelling is predominant.

After *Apis* or even without passing through the stage of *Apis* the patient may come to the field of *Mercurius solubilis*.

Often the rheumatism is aggravated at night. The patient has frequent sweats, oily, bad smelling sweat. The mouth is mist but no thirst.

After *Mercurius* you have the stage of *Pulsatilla* and of *Silicea*. If the patient has suppurations he enters into the stage of *Hepar sulphur*. *Pulsatilla* and *Silicea* often indicate venous congestion, amelioration and finally cure. At this time you can use *Sulphur* to check periodical relapse.

The chronic rheumatic patient may follow two paths. That of the digestive and hepatic troubles and that of periodic attack of acute or subacute rheumatism.

The other groups are related to *Lycopodium*, *Natrum sulphuricum*, and *Thuja*.

Lycopodium has a kind of acid diathesis which is related to dehydration of albuminoids. Thus it has as complementaries the salts of *Lithium* : The *Corbonate*, the *Benzoate*, *Benzoic acid* and also *Ammonium benzoicum*, a group of four remedies which may act as complementaries of *Thuja*, but they are at that stage complementaries of *Lycopodium*. If you use these remedies empirically and not in *Lycopodium* subjects you will get only inconstant results. They act better in lower dilutions and in ponderable doses. The high indilutions are generally inefficacious. *Sarsaparilla* and *Kali carbonicum* may be placed in this group.

The hydrogenoid group is more homogeneous, and most easy to manipulate. The most important are *Rhus tox* and *Dulcamara* which are drainers of *Natrum sulphuricum* and *Thuja*. The subject has the need of being drained by *Rhus tox* (which acts better when applied in the morning) by *Rhus radicans* or any other *Rhus*. *Rododendron* is aggravated by cold and in humid weather. *Rhus tox* is one of the most unfaithful remedies, it often fails. When it fails *Rododendron* may be used. Perhaps we do not know well the application of the dilutions of *Rhus tox* or its preparation is not from fresh plant. It is always difficult to have an active *Rhus*.

Dulcamara is aggravated by humidity or in summer after having suddenly taken cold or having seated on a humid place. *Ranunculus bulbosus* has, like *Rhus tox*, some cutaneous affections, eczema or neuralgia or rheumatic pains of the intercostal spaces. *Aranea diadema* is a typical drainer of all hydrogenoids specially of *Natrum sulphuricum* types; you may use it in 3x in *Natrum sulphuricum* subjects with *Rhus tox 30*.

We must not forget that there are other drainers of hydrogenoid state. I cannot indicate all of them here. As for example *Nux vomica* and *Ipecac* are often very good drainers in these cases. *Ammonium causticum* may be related to *Aranea diadema*. The patient is weak, and worn out.

Let us now pass to the compounds of *Iodide*. It is certain that in allopathy *Iodium* gives good results in some forms of rheumatism. I think that when we use *Plumbum iodatum, Natrum iodatum, Kali iodatum* in lower dilutions we somewhat behave like the allopaths without knowing it. Similarly the allopaths sometimes do homoeopathy without knowing it. The most important of these remedies is *Kali iodatum* which is a remedy of syphilitic condition.

There is another group of remedies, which goes out of our field. They are remedies of neuralgia. These remedies are to be given to persons having hybrid pains, neuralgic as well as rheumatic pains. It is the group headed by *Kalmia, Guaicum* etc.

Kalmia is used in the rheumatism of upper limbs. *Ledum palustre* is used in the rheumatism of the lower limbs. *Kalmia* is very erratic, it has fulgurating pains. In *Ledum palustre* the pains go from above downwards.

Guaicum is related to *Thuja* and to all remedies that act on the rheumatic pains and at the same time on kidneys. When *Rhus tox* or *Dulcamara* do not act you may use this remedy specially when the neuralgia is alternated with numbness.

Derris pinata was indicated to me by Dr. Cartier who insists on three remedies which are less known.

Radium Bromide is used in homoeopathy in the same manner as it is used in allopathy as radium pommades, which act well in rheumatic patients. It is a good remedy but sometimes aggravate. It must be given in high dilutions. *Magnesia carbonic* is to be used in patients suffering from neuralgia who has some very acute pains. The patient cannot bear the pains like that of *Chamomilla*; he is hypersensitive. These patients have pains at the roots of hairs. *Oxalic acid* is interesting in chronic rheumatism. The patients have atrocious pains with neuralgia, neuritis and some phenomena that may lead us to think of myelitis.

In relation to *Silicea* we must think of all the remedies acting on rheumatism of bones. *Ruta* acts specially on cartilages and has the sensation as if the pains are from a bruise. In all affections of bones you will find syphilis as a cause. I insist on the value of *Phytolacca*. It is to be given repeatedly in 3x. I only mention here the other remedies : *Mezereum, Kali bichromicum, Kali iodatum, Stillingia, Mercurius, Aurum.* I often use *Silicea* 200 followed by *Ruta* 30, *Arnica* 30, *Phytolacca* 3x.

With *Pulsatilla* we have the remedies of venous and capillary congestion and circulatory troubles. It is a very important remedy. The group of remedies having erratic pains is related to it and *Stellaria* is related to circulatory troubles. *Kali bichromicum, Lac canimum, Kali sulphuricum* are complementaries of *Pulsatilla* and have like it erratic pains. *Colchicum, Ferrum metallicum,* and *Sangunaria* are not erratic. I have indicated them here because they have circulatory troubles. *Colchicum* is a remedy of gout, the pericardia is affected by this remedy. *Ferrum metallicum* is a remedy of anemia and rheumatism of the left shoulder whereas *Sangunaria* is a remedy of the rheumatism of the right shoulder.

Finally you have *Cimicifuga* a remedy of muscular rheumatism. The first remedy of this group is *Arnica*, which has contusions and muscular pains. *Lac canimum* was a patient of *Lachesis* who has passed into the field of *Cimicifuga*. *Lac canimum* is an excellent remedy of rheumatism with neuralgia and pains coming during menopause. *Caulophyllum* is a good remedy to open a recalcitrant *col uteri*. It is marvellous for the muscles of the sphinisters. *Actea spicata* is a very important remedy of rheumatism of small joints.

Colocynthis has cramps coming out of cold, better by bending double. *Agaricus* has spasms, cramps and muscular jerkings. *Rananculus bulbosus, Bryonia* and *Lachnanthes* act on torticolis and vertebral rheumatism.

Ground remedies of secondary importance are *Nux vomica* in relation to *Sulphur* ; *Graphitis* is related to *Calcarea carbonica* ; *Arsenicum album* is related to *Lycopodium* ; *Iodium* is related to *Cimicifuga*, but these remedies are less important.

There are great many more remedies that we could have indicated, but to be more practical we have limited ourselves only to the principal remedies.

SYMPTOMATOLOGY OF THE REMEDIES OF RHEUMATISM

Basic Remedies :

Phosphorus—This remedy has particular affinity to the tissues. For this reason its field in rheumatism is very wide.

Its pathogenesis is not yet well known but its Homoeopathic application must be very wide. It is Dr. Bernoville who says that this remedy is to be tried in old sclerous rheumatic patients, having tendency ankylosis.

Its symptoms are : The patient is generally old, having tendency to sclerosis ; he is of syphilitic type. Feet are cold ; hands hot or burning. Pulse often rapid. Head is easily congested ; tendency to vertigo. Desire for cold drinks. Great sensitiveness to change of weather, specially to stormy weather.

The 200th potency is used at an interval of 20 to 30 days according to the reappearance of the symptoms.

Its marked effects on pains as well as on the general condition of the patient have led us to think that in the treatment of chronic rheumatism, this remedy will be necessary at one time or another.

Sulphur—We are going to give here only some characteristics of this remedy which are seen in chronic rheumatism.

(*a*) Chilly patient, eats less, has itching of the skin with or without eruption. Feet are cold, head is hot. The articulations are stiff and crackling. Drawning and burning pains in the evening or at night, during change of weather. *Hyperthyroidian* patient. In this case *Sulphur* is used in decimals, frequently repeated with Thyroid which is given in ponderable doses.

(*b*) The patient is always very hot, with the feet burning. Congestion of the face, lips and ears are red. Hunger and thirst, goneness feeling in the stomach at 11 A.M., morning diarrhoea. Itching at night in the heat of the bed.

The rheumatic affections are not so much stubborn as in the first type. Use *Sulphur* 200. A few doses will soon give good results.

Thuya—It is an antisycotic remedy. It is very often indicated when there is the history of gonorrhoea. Here it is complementary to *Medorrhinum*. But for its use one should depend on its totality of symptoms even when there is no history of gonorrhoea.

Its characteristics are :

Aggr. Cold damp weather. It can be compared with *Natrum sulphuricum, Rhus tox* and *Dulcamara.*

A left sided remedy. Aggr. 3 to 4 a.m.

Articular pains worse during rest. The patient must move when he is on bed. If he is not sycotic, says Kent, *Rhus tox* will cure him, but when sycosis is intricated in the case *Thuya* or *Medorrhinum* will be necessary to complete the cure, specially when the symptoms appear after the suppression of gonorrhoea. Dark persons with black hair, corpulont, having a big belly, thick skin, greasy, with accentuated features. Varicose veins of the nose ; Localised sweats of the uncovered parts. Particularly the soles of the feet are sensitive (*Medorrhinum*).

Tendency to growths (cauli flower growth, condylomes, naeve). Action of *Thuya* should be completed by *Medorrhinum* or T.R. Afterwards the symptoms of *Sulphur* will appear.

Lycopodium—*Lycopodium* is an auto-intoxicated, sedentary type, whose liver does not work well. Urecimic, later on uremic persons.

It has *Calcium* and *Uric acid* deposits on joints.

Persons with emaciated thorax, limbs have weak muscles, with the face like that of an old man, having transverse frontal wrinkles ; yellow spots on the temples ; slow digestion of farinaceous foods ; somnolence after meals with distention of the stomach ; vertigo, loss of memory.

Aggr. of all symptoms between 4 and 8 p.m.

Drawing, tearing pains aggravated by hot applications.

Amel. by light movements. Desire for constant movement of an arm or of a leg. One foot cold the other hot.

Specially the elbows and the small joints are affected (compare *Medorrhinum, Caulophyllus, Actea spicata, Kali bichromicum, Natrum phos, Ruta*).

Red sand deposit in the urine. The general condition becomes good after this deposit.

At the beginning of the treatment lower dilutions are necessary because a high dilution may block the liver and may cause congestion. The drainer of *Lycopodium* are *Chelidonium*, *Carduus marianus Taraxacum* (in decimals).

The articular drainers are *Bryonia*, *Rhus tox*, *Argentum nitricum*, etc.

Bryonia—It is an important remedy of synovitis (*Apis*, *Cantharis*). It will be frequently indicated.

Its characteristics are very clear. Stinging pains in joints, very sensitive to pressure (by tips of a finger, but better by wide pressure by palms). This characteristic is marked in acute cases when there is strong effusion. However, it is used in chronic cases.

· Articular serous inflammation explains the characteristic of the remedy : Aggravation by the least movement. Aggravation by continuous movement. The patient tries to remain completely immobile. The pains are generally fixed and is slightly ameliorated by local heat.

It is opposite of *Rhus tox*, which is a remedy of peri-articular tissue.

Teste speaks of a *Bryonia* type with firm flesh, accustomed to rich food. Kent speaks of a gouty type having renal troubles. Others describe *Bryonia* as a lean, dark, subject with bilious colour of the skin. Clarke says that because of its very wide action we should not look for a definite type.

The chronic type of *Bryonia* seems to be an auto-intoxicated of whose the liver and the kidneys do not function well. He cannot bear prolonged physical fatigue and excess of dishes. Generally it is a remedy of serouses. It is related to *Lycopodium, Oxalic acid, Rhus tox.*

Rhus Toxicodendorn – It is a remedy of fibrous tissues (*Ruta, Phytolacca, Rhododendron*). The modalities are important : Aggr. by rest and by the first movement. Amel. by continued movement.

It is complementary to *Bryonia*. There is alternation of symptoms to these two remedies.

Amel. by heat and Aggr. by cold and damp weather.

Compare with *Kali iodatum* which has aggr. by movement. But *Rhus tox* is chilly and wants heat and is easily fatigued. *Kali iod* wants cold, and bears exercises without marked fatigue.

Causticum—According to Nash, *Sulphur, Rhus tox* and *Causticum* are frequently indicated in chronic rheumatism.

Its symptoms are almost similar to those of *Rhus tox.* They are to be distinguished. *Rhus tox* is continually in movement, while *Causticum* is agitated only at night ; movement does not ameliorate his pains.

Rhus tox has amelioration in cold and humid weather while *Causticum* is aggravated in dry weather and particularly in dry cold weather. It is a remedy of tendons which have a tendency to become retracted. The joints are stiff, painful movement with the sensation of being scorched. In

Causticum there is often a great weakness with a tendency to paresis and trembling. 12th and 30th dilutions are generally suitable.

Argentum Nitricum—We have often seen the rapidity of the action of this remedy on pains as well as on functional troubles. In our observations we apply it on the following symptoms :

Stinging pains as if from splinters, but we have also seen that even when this symptom does not exist, there is often very rapid amelioration.

Frequent modalities are : Aggr. by the first movement even when continued ; Amel. by heat, by wide pressure.

Associated but not constant symptoms : Desire for sugar ; tired look, often seems older than his age. The symptoms are associated with those of *Lycopodium* and *Arsenicum album*.

This remedy generally acts on lumbo-sacral pains and on pains of small joints and big joints. It seems that this remedy has affinity to synovial as well as on peri-articular tissues.

The rapidity and persistent action of this remedy used in different case have led us to think that though this remedy has not well characterised modalities yet it should be one of the important remedies of chronic rheumatism.

Other Remedies :

Actaea Racemosa (Cimicifuga)—Muscular rheumatism. Aggravation of all symptoms during menses (inverse-*Lachesis*). Often used in pains of menopause.

Apis—Chronic rheumatism with or without exudation. Aggr. by heat ; Amel. by cold application. Sharp stinging pains.

Local hypersensitiveness—Absence of thirst (*Apis 200*).

Amel. by cold applications. Compare : Cantharis and the serpent poisons.

Benzoic Acid—Rheumatism related to the infection of urinary tract : colibacilosis or other. Strong repulsive odour of the urine. Very great pain in the renal region. Articular pains aggr. by movement. Pains of tendon Achilles (*Ruta*).

Berberis Vulgaris—Erratic gouty rheumatism. Charged urine. Cutting and beating pains in the renal region (left), irradiating to the thigh. Hepatic troubles, with sensitive vesicular point.

Calcarea Fluorica—Complementary *Rhus tox* by its affinity to fibrous peri-articular tissue ; its aggravation by rest, by cold and by humid weather, its amelioration by heat and movement. Heredo type, Malcunction of the pituitary.

Calcarea Phos—Rheumatism of small joints. Rapidly changes place. Amel. of pains by closing hands. Concomittant uterine troubles.

Colchicum—Gouty rheumatism ; erratic pains, extremely painful ; Aggr. at night and by movement. Affinity to toes. Hypersensitiveness with great weakness. Intolerence of smells. Distended abdomen.

Dulcamara—Articular pains, aggr. by change of weather (humid weather). The modalities are similar to those of *Rhus tox*. It is often an acute of *Natrum Sulf*.

Elaps Carolinus—Patient suffers from obesity, congestion, hypertention. Somnolence. Gouty modalities. Strong elimination of *Uric acid* in the urine. Diabetis.

General symptoms are similar to those of *Lachesis* (gushes of heat, desire for fresh air, aggr. after sleep). Generally *30th potency* is used.

Formica Rufa—Rheumatic troubles related to a renal infection (colibacilocis). Bad smell of the urine, pyuria. Burning erratic pain, aggr. by movement, cold application, before snowfall. Amel. by heat, by rubbing, after midnight, Profuse sweat that does not ameliorate.

Kali Bichromicum—Acute pains, rapidly shifting from one joint to the other (*Lac caninum, Kali sulph, Manganum, Pulsatilla. Stellaria* media). Pains appear and disappear rapidly (Phytolacca).

Alter rheumatic and digestive troubles. Affinity to small joints (*Caulophyllum, Ledum, Lycopodium, Medorrhinum, Ruta*).

Sensitiveness of bones (particularly of tibia). Heels are sensitive. Aggr. by night and by cold.

Kali Iodatum—A remedy having affinity to fibrous tissue and periosteum. Pasty swelling of articulations (particularly of the knee). Bone pains. Tibia sensitive to touch. Rheumatisms with pains worse at night, by immobility. Gouty old persons, must move ceaselessly, wants open air, and have great heat. Fatigue when remains immobile and suffers much : he can walk for a long time in the open air without fatigue, specially when the weather is cold.

Kalmia— Rheumatic spasms from above downwards (inverse *Ledum*). Fleeting lightning like pains, erratic pains. Heart troubles of the gout, with acute pains in the heart. Slow pulse.

Lac Caninum—Great shifting of pains from left to right or right to left.

Ledum—Ascending rheumatism. Localised on feet, soles are sensitive (*Antimonium crudum, Medorrhinum, Thuya, Natrum sulph*). The patient is particularly chilly but his rheumatic pains are ameliorated while bathing in cold water and the heat of the bed aggravates the pains.

Natrum Muriaticum—It gives good results in rheumatism of persons living on sea-side and when other remedies have failed. It is used in 6x or 12x.

Natrum Sulphuricum—Auto-intoxicated persons suffering from insufficient function of the liver and retention of water, having tendency to obesity, having periodic morning diarrhoea. Insufficient function of glands. Aggr. by humidity (by all sorts of humid atmospheres). Amel. in hot and dry atmosphere. Periodic asthma and skin troubles. Different articular pains ; aggr. by rest, in humid weather soles of the feet are very sensitive, some times with burning sensation.

Complementary : *Arania, Arsenic alb., Dulcamara, Rhus tox, Thuya.*

Petroleum—Stiff and painful articulations ; crackling. Sensation of localised coldness. Burning of hands and feet that the patient puts out of the bed. Aggr. in winter by change of weather, in cold air. Amel. in summer. Dry, rough skin, easily cracks, specially in the winter season. Itching Gastric troubles. *Petroleum* is often indicated in chronic gonorrhoeal catarrh and it is used in arthritis of gonorrhoeal origin.

Phytolacca—Affinity to fibrous tissue and periosteum. Erractic panis coming and going suddenly like electric shocks (*Kalmia, Kali bichromicum*). The patient is very much undown tries to find amelioration by movement. Aggr. at night and in humid weather. Osteocopic pains ; pains of the heels (Talalgia). Sciatic pains. Syphilitic ground.

Pulsatilla—The pain moves rapidly from one place to another. Aggr. in the evening, by rest, by heat. Amel. by movement, by open air. Absence of thirst.

Rhododendron—Aggr. In windy or stormy weather is the most important characteristic Amel. by movement. Rheumatic gout.

Ruta—Affinity to bone tissues, cartilages and fibrous tissues. Aggr. by rest, humidity at night. Rheumatism of small articulations. Pains of the tendon Achille.

Silicea—Advanced stage of sclerosis is very chilly old persons. Nails are yellow, breaking, deformed. Sensitiveness of the soles.

Nosodes :

Medorrhinum—Chronic, rebellious, gouty rheumatic affection. Rheumatism, neuralgia, myelitis and it is used when other remedies do not act. Aggr. during the day (from sunrise to sun set), by movement, when the patient thinks about the aggravation (*Oxalic acid, Helonias, Ignatia*), by heat, and during storm. Amel. by humid weather (*Causticum*, *Nux vomica*). Affinity to small articulations. Erratic pains coming and going suddenly. Movements of the feet at night. Hands and feet burns at night (*Sulphur*, *Petroleum*). Hasty patients (*Argentum nit.*), loss of memory.

Complementaries : *Natrum sulph.*, *Thuya*, *T.R.*, *Rhus tox. T.R.* (Residual Tuberculin of Koch).

Chronic cases with tuberculous heridity, Aggr. by rest, by the first movement, in cold and humid weather. Amel. by local heat, by continued movement. In a word the symptoms of *Rhus tox*, which *Rhus tox* cannot alone cure.

Frequent complementary : *Sulphur*, *Thuya*, *Rhus tox*, *Luesinum* (*Syphilinum*).

Aggr. at night (from sunset to sunrise), by humid weather. Amel. during the day, on mountains. Aggravation and amelioration are always progressive. Pains of bones. Headache, Alopecia. Profuse salivation.

Amel. during the day, on mountain.

Aggravation and Amelioration are always progressive. Pains of bones. Headache. Alopecia. Profuse salivation.

Acute Articular Rheumatism :

Considered as a specific and autonomous disease, although the pathogenic agent is still unknown, acute articular rheumatism requires a deep study from the Homoeopathic point of view. The conception about acute articular rheumatism is sensibly different to the idea which has led to give the name of this disease : Bouilland's disease.

According to the modern authors the joints are hardly attacked or less attacked and that the articular rheumatism is not a disease of the articulations but a general disease which can be defined as chronic cardiopathy complicated with fluxional inflammation of the articular serouses. The infection seems to act specially to persons of oxygenoid tuberculitic type of *Natrum Sulphuricum, Sulphur Iodatum, Calcarea* or *Kali Carbonicum*. Its periodicity seems to be annual which is predominantly *Phosphorus* and those that come in July or August are predominantly *Sulphur*.

Finally let me say that there is a possible relation with chorea and acute articular rheumatism, but let me also say that the nature of chorea is also still obscure as that of the acute articular rheumatism. The relation between the two affections are very much controversial.

The possibility of co-existence of the alternate choreic movement and rheumatic arthralgia is undeniable. Charcot says that chorea and rheumatism are two distinct diseases and rheumatism would only play the part of determining agent like all other infectious diseases, for the apparition of chorea.

On the contrary, for all the pediatrics chorea is essentially a real rheumatism and in infants it is similar to the cerebral rheumatism of the adult. Fraenkel has besides shown the existence of Aschoff nodules in chronic myocardia. Clinic shows frequent articular attacks in course of a choreic attack or their alternance.

Finally let us study the Homoeopathic treatment of acute articular rheumatism.

(A) Beginning. *Angina*—Ordinary red inflammation exists in one third of the cases with some mild functional symptoms and therefore rarely treated except in cases where it coincides with arthritis.

Aconite—Dry skin, agitation, anxiety, thirst. Attack after exposure to dry cold. Used in lower dilutions (1x to 3x and even M.T.)

Ferrum Phosphoricum—(3x to 6x) Less intense fever than that of *Aconite*. Sweat. Soft pulse. It is a link to *Belladonna* : throbbing sweat, mydriasis.

Mercurius Solubilis—Attack comes after cold at night. Night sweat without relief. Humid tongue, gray coating, imprint of teeth. Salivation, breath and sweat have foul smell. Then comes the stage when the disease is established. In this stage the medicines already described are useful and the disease may be checked.

(B) The disease is established. *Bryonia* (1x to 6x)—A remedy of serous membranes in opposition to *Rhus tox* which attacks the peri-articular tissue. It has action on temporo-maxiller joint.

Bryonia—It is characterised by its stinging acute pain. The patient remains immobile. Great thirst with dry mouth. Pains ameliorate by cold application and by wide pressure (by the palm).

Rhus Toxicodendron—The modalities are inverse. Agitation, aggr. at night. Red triangle on the tip of the tongue. *Bryonia* and *Rhus tox* succeed each other more often.

than they oppose each other. *Rhus tox* will be specially indicated in a dynamic state.

Apis (3x to 6)—Erratic pains, not so severe. Absence of thirst. Stinging and burning pains, worse by cold application, amel. by cold. Absence of thirst. When there is renal lesions this remedy is to be thought of.

Pulsatilla (3x to 6)—Erratic pains, not so severe. Absence of thirst. Chilliness.

Lac Canimum—It is not so important, but it is to be used with *Pulsatilla*. Pains alternating from one side to the other.

Chamomilla (3x to 6)—Used in acute articular rheumatism of children. Very great pain, patient cannot bear it. Irritability. One cheek more red than the other.

Kali Bichromicum—Erratic pains on some fixed places which may be covered by the finger tip.

Benzoic Acid (3x to 6) —Strong urine with strong smell of amonia.

Colchicum—Sub-actue stage. Symptoms of *Bryonia* but the general condition is more serious. Sensitiveness to outward impressions, to noise and to light.

Cantharis—It will be indicated only when there is pleural localisation.

Sodium Salicilate—It may be used in small doses 1/1000 every two hours. In the pathogenesis of *Salicylic acid* Boericke writes : Articular attack with stinging pains, aggr. by touch, movement. Profuse sweat does not ameliorates (Merc sol).

Burning of the stomach, vertigo. **Temporary Deafness**.

Dose : 3x, repeated every three hours.

Veratrum Album—Grave adynamic form.   Delirium.

End :

At this stage we often find the indications of *Sulphur* 30 (In Oxygenoid type it is preferable to give *Sulphur iodatum*). Heat in the top of the head with cold feet.   Jerkings of the arms while sleeping.

Natrum Muriaticum (200)—Weeping look.   Marked anemia.   Pale mucous membranes.   Goneness feeling in the stomach towards 10 A.M.

Natrum Muriaticum is indicated when there is trouble of metabolism of salt and troubles caused by the abuse of *Salycilate*.

Natrum Muriaticum is complementary of *Ferrum Metallicum*, *Pulsatilla* and *China* 6.

Marmoreck 30, Spengler or Aviary in tuberculinics, always observing the rules for the use of tuberculins.

These remedies of convalescence : *Natrum Muriaticum*, *Sulphur iod.* and the tuberculins are to be well drained by *China* 6, *Kali Phos* 6 *Silicea* 30 and *Avena Sativa* 1x.

Cardiac Localisation :

From the beginning when symptoms of *Ferrum Phos* are seen one must think of Cardiac localisation.   Then very rapidly the following remedies are to be added to the treatment of cardiac localisation. *Spigelia* 6. Dyspnoea with anxiety (myocardia is affected). Constricting sensation (*Cactus*). Aggr. after sleep (*Lachesis*).

If the condition aggravates :

Arsenicum Album (6)—Great anxiety. Fear of death. Dyspnoea aggravates at night from midnight to 3 A.M. Tongue as if roasted. Thirst for small quantities of water repeatedly.

Pyrogenium—It should be given before the clinical indications. *Echinacea M.T.* May be used even intraveinously.

Streptococcin :

Some other remedies are those that we have already been studied.

Apis—Stinging pain in the region of heart. Partial oedema. No thirst. Aggr. by heat.

Bryonia—Dry cough, painful. Cardiac pains. Better when the patient lies on the left side (pericarditis). Dry mouth. Great thirst.

Rhus Toxicodendron—Complementary to Bryonia. Agitation. Pain all over the body.

Kalmia (*3x to 6x*)—Lightning like pains, rapidly change places, and irradiate below (inverse of ledum). Slow pulse. Alternance of cardiac symptoms and rheumatic symptoms.

Aurum Metallicum—Very tumultuous beating of the heart. Dyspnoea while sitting down or bending forward.

The development of articular rheumatism in tuberculinic and oxygenoid subjects explains the relative frequency of pleuropulmonary complications, either congestion of the lungs or rheumatic pleurisy.

Classical rheumatic pleurisy of Lasigne type sometimes bilateral will require *Bryonia* and *Cantharis*.

Convalescence.

In order to avoid sequalae of acute articular rheumatism : *Natrum Muriaticum, Sulphur iodatum* and *Tuberculins* in high dilutions. Sometimes *Thuya 200, Baryta Muriaticum 200* and *Rheumatoxin*, a nosode obtained from a drop of blood of a rheumatic patient, and diluted, which is given alternately with the ground remedies and Tuberculins.

Thus we will be able to check the terrible Osler's disease and the evolution of cardiac rheumatism.

SCIATICA

Sciatica is a very well known affection. Its definition can be found in any pathological treatise, so we do not make an attempt to define it. We insist only that one should not make errors of diagnosis. Our therapeutic study is only for essential and old sciatica which the doctors should not confound with secondary or symptomatic sciatica. If the clinic is not sufficient the doctor must try to diagonose it by all means, by radiography by lumber puncture etc. We have not divided our study into chronic and acute forms. The same medicine may suit to both the cases. We have given only those symptoms of the remedies that correspond particularly to both acute and chronic sciatica. We are not discussing here the question of pathology and etiology, not because we ignore their importance but because the study of the ground will help us to deduce naturally the answer to those questions.

Our friends will excuse us for the long list of remedies. We have tried to be complete but it is possible that we may have left out some of the medicines.

1. Morbid Ground :

The knowledge of the ground is an essential factor for the sure success of the treatment.

In simple cases the medicines symptomatically used may alone cure the pains but in stubborn cases constitutional remedies are to be added to them. The constitutional remedies will be very frequently indispensable to avoid relapse. On what grounds sciatica develops :

(1) Sycotic ground is the most important of all. The subjects are mostly hydrogenoids, sensitive to humidity and to variations Aggr. While standing. At night, by the heat of the bed, by rest (need for movement). Amel. moving the feet, to find a cold place, by moderate walking. Piercing, drawing pains with heaviness, numbness from hip to foot.

General : Horror of washing. Goneness feeling in the stomach at 11 A.M. Burning feet, Morning diarrhoea. Cutaneous eruptions.

Thuya (200, M)—Sycosis. Hydrogenoid.

Left sided (non-exclusive) Aggr. by immobility, on bed, by humidity. Amel. while moving constantly moving. Drawing pain along the nerve, in the soles.

General : Obsessions. Fixed ideas. Lower lip bluish-white. Sweat of uncovered parts. Genito-urinary affections. Tendency to proliferations (warts etc.).

Let us then study eight remedies with their indications :

(1) *Cimicifuga* (30, 200, M)—With the preceding it is one of the most important of ground remedies of sciatica. It is useful in rheumatoid pains having a particular affinity to long muscles on which because of its spasmophile tendency, it processes cramps. Left sided. Aggr. while lying down ; should go out of bed. During menses. Amel. by continued movement, by pressure. In open air. Violent pains with anxiety in legs. Heaviness. Incessant agitation of the lower limbs cramps. Uteroovarian troubles. Irritability. Fear of becoming mad. Hysteria.

(2) *Lycopodium* (6, 30, 200, M)—Insufficient liver. Carbonitrogenoid. Cancer state. Indifferent laterality (more right sided). Aggr. by rest, in bed, lying on the painful side, while standing, Amel. by movement.

Chronic Sciatica, periodic with remission. Pains after every **four** days. Weakness and stiffness of the limbs. Cannot stretch the leg. Bad digestion. Face like an old man. Big belly and lean limbs. Horror of solitude. Aggr. from 5 to 8 P.M.

(3) *Lachesis* (12, 30, 200, M)—Endocrinal intoxication, menopause, alcoholism. Indifferent laterality, Pain going from left to right. Aggr. after sleep, standing, by movement, by contact. Amel. by menstruation, by discharges, while lying down, by hot application. Burning pain along the

nerve. Loquacity. Jealousy. Gushes of heat. Alternate excitation and depression. Bad effect of solar heat.

(4) *Nux Vomica* (6, 30, 200, M)—Hepatic insufficiency. Digestive intoxication. All sorts of abuses. Indifferent laterality. Aggr. by movement. In the morning (4 to 5 A.M.), by cold. Amel. by rest, hot application. Tearing pain from above downwards with spasm. Jerkings of muscles, contractions, stiffness. Sensation as if the limbs are paralysed. Abuse of stimulants. Excess of sedentarism. Business cares. Irritability. General amel. by wet and mild climate.

(5) *Natrum Sulphuricum* (200, M)—Hydrogenoid. Rheumatism. Congestion of liver. Indifferent laterality (more left sided). Aggr. by all forms of humidity. Lying on the left side. Abuse of quinine. Amel. by dry weather, by pressure, change of position. Disgust of life. Tendency to suicide. Flatulence, thirst, morning diarrhoea. Inflammation of fingers around nails.

(6) *Ignatia* (30, 200, M)—Intoxication reflecting on nerves. Results of grief and cares. Indifferent laterality (more left sided). Aggr. by change of position, standing, by walking. At night, in open air. After eating, by coffee and tobacco. Amel. by rest, by lying down, during eating. Pains with spasms, intense, stiffness, cutting pains in the hips. Sensation as if coxofemoral articulation is broken. A remedy of women. Physical and mental hypertension. Paradoxal alternance of gaity and sadness. Contradictory symptoms. Never speak about her ennuies.

(7) *Causticum* (6, 30, 200)—Hydrogenoid. Chronic rheumatism. Indifferent laterality. Aggr. by temperate humid

weather. Heat of the bed, by heat. Numbness and agitations of limbs. Heavyness, weakness, tremblings. Sensation as if **the tendons are very short**. Chronic rheumatism with crushing pain on the articulations. Sensitiveness for others. Fear of darkness. Sensation of an open sore.

(8) *Sepia* (30, 2000, M)—Hepatic insufficiency. Genital affections. Tuberculinism. Indifferent laterality (more left side). Aggr. in the morning and in the evening, by humidity and in cold. Amel. by violent exercise, by heat. Weakness and agitation, heavyness of the limbs. Sadness. Indifference. Aggr. by consolation. Bearing down. Cannot lie on the left side.

Let us cite here four other remedies that are less frequently used: *Calcarea Carbonica* (Psora, **Sciatica after working in water**) of temperature. In the antecedents we find gonorrhoea, vaccination or serological injections.

(1) Two ground remedies are useful : *Thuya* and *Natrum Sulphuricum*. The first one is more important than the second one. The nosode Medorrhinum will give good result.

(2) Psora ground which arthritism is one of the aspect is very favourable for sciatica : *Sulphur* and *Psorinum* are the ground remedies, the first one is more important than the second. If there is the doubt that tuberculosis is closely connected with *Psora*, *Marmoreck* and *T.R.* should be used in oxygenoids and *T.R.* in hydrogenoids. These will be the remedies.

(3) For syphilitic ground *Luesinum* is to be used.

(4) The cancer ground, with its deep intoxication, its eliminations or its fixations along a nerve is also a cause of

sciatica. The ground remedies such as *Lycopodium, Arseni-cum* should be carefully individualised because of the morbid transfer. The most recommendable nosode is heterogenous or autogenous Sanguin therapy (isopathy).

Finally we should recommend not to omit in the interrogatory an enquiry on possible traumatism :

2. Ground Remedies. We are first of all taking up the study of some remedies that we consider particularly are remedies of the ground of Sciatica but, if they cover well the cause, may also be used as spmptomatic remedies. When they are used as ground remedies, they are to be prescribed in high dilutions (200, M) ; on the contrary in 6 and 30. The most important are *Sulphur* and *Thuya*.

Sulphur (30, 200, M.) Psora. Left sided. *Graphites* (Psora, chilliness), *Natrum Muriaticum* (tuberculinics, Aggar. on sea side) and *Silicea* (tuberculinics, extreme sensitiveness to cold) and we will add two nosodes : *Medorrhinum* and *Luesinum.*

Medorrhinum (200, M)—Indifferent laterality. Aggr. of all symptoms while thinking about them. Amel. on sea side, at night. Changing character impatient, anxious. Time passes very slowly. Fear of becoming mad. Sensation of heat ; burning pains in the brain ; sweating palms. Feels her uterus (Dr. Chiron) ; bad smell of the skin, of secretions.

Luesinum (200, M)—Indifferent laterality. Aggr. at night on sea side. Amel. on mountains. Excessive nervousness, anxious for his health, diminution of memory. Continually washed his hands, desire for alcohol. Pains increases and decreases gradually. Bone pains. Headache. Deep longitudinal crack of the tongue (Dr. Chiron). Agitation of the limbs which he must move continually. In sciatica movement and walking ameliorate.

Considered as ground remedies, they should be used in high dilutions (200, M) and should be repeated at long intervals (three weeks or one month).

3. Symptomatic Remedies. In sciatica if one wants to be successful he must look for "Simile" or "Similimum". The result will be as favourable as the medicines are individualised. Two remedies repeated alternately, at an interval of two to three hours, when more than one remedies are chosen. In chronic cases 6 or 30, once or twice. When there is the possibility of finding a single remedy it is then the triumph of Unicism and in that case the medicine may be used according to the Kentian fashion, in high dilution waiting for the results.

We have classified the remedies in three groups : At first three most important remedies, then remedies in alphabetical order, which are frequently used, and finally the exceptionally or rarely indicated remedies.

A. *Bryonia* (6, 30)—Indifferent laterality. Aggr. by movement, while standing, by superficial contact. Amel. by rest, lying on the affected side, by strong pressure. Drawing pains, lancinating as if from a "sore below the skin", of which the seat is on the lumber region and on hips. General aggr. by heat, anger. Dryness of the muscous membranes with thirst for large quantities of water at long intervals. Constipation.

Gnaphallium (6, 30)—Indifferent laterality. Aggr. by walking, by movement, however feels the necessity of movement and change of position ; while lying down. Amel. while sitting, bending the legs. Intense pains, ccntinued pains alternating with numbness. Cramp of the calfs and hips. Foetid diarrhoea, with colic, aggr. in the morning.

Kali bicaromicum (6, 30)—Left side. Aggr. while standing sitttting lying down (must change position). Amel. by walking, by flexion of limbs. Violent pain, moving along a limb ; appearing and disappearing suddenly. General aggr. by cold, humid coldness ; towards or three A.M. Aggr. by drinking beier.

B. Remedies Having Frequent Indications :

Aconite (6, 30)—Indifferent laterality. Agg. at night, by movement, by the heat of the room. Amel. by rest and while sitting. Acute sciatica. Sudden attack after being exposed to dry cold. Extreme physical and mental agitation. Intolerance of heat. Fear of death. Hypersensitiveness to contact. Pain with numbness.

Ammonium Muriaticum (6, 30)—Left sided. Aggr. while sitting down. Slight amelioration while walking, complete while lying down. Chronic Sciatica. Sometimes grave from, with tearing pains, stinging pains accompanied by contraction of the limb which causes limping. Menses abundant at night.

Arnica (6, 30)—Indifferent laterality. Agg. in the evening, at night, by movement. (Should change position), by coldness. Amel while. lying down. Burning, tearing pains.

Traumatic sensation, sensation of fracture, numbness. Traumatic sciatica. Creates a scene when the doctor arrives, does not require his service.

Arsenicum Album (6, 30, 200)—Indifferent laterality. Aggr. at night from midnight to 2 A.M., by cold and cold application by violent movement. Amel. by heat and hot applications. Burning and tearing pains forcing the patient to constantly change position. Prefers to lie down but constantly moves. Agitation, weakness. Fear of death. Refuses to take medicines because he is hopeless of cure.

Belladonna (6, 30)—Indifferent laterality. Aggr. at night, after midnight. By touch, by the least contact, by sound and light, by gush of wind. Amel. while standing, hanging the affected limb ; by half sitting position, by heat. Pains appearing and disappearing suddenly. Periodical attack, beginning in the afternoon and ending at midnight. Alternate agitation and depression. Hyperesthesia of senses. Tendency to spasms. Dilatation of pupils.

Bufo (6, 30)—Indifferent laterality. Aggr. by heat. In a hot room, during sleep. Amel. by haemorrhage, by putting the feet in hot water. Mental weakness, idiocy in depressed persons, as a result of sexual abuse or of onanism. Sudden anger, bites. Epilepsy.

Chamomilla (6, 30)—Left laterality (non-exclusive). Aggr. at night, in bed, by the least movement, by rest. Amel. when carried, being a vehicle. Slight amel. by cold. Pain with numbness. Intolerance of pains, with great agitations, cries, tendency to become angry. Need for movement when suffering. General aggravation by anger and fear. General amel. by humid heat.

Cocculus (6,30)—Indifferent laterality. Aggr. by contact, by noise, in open air, afternoon. Amel. by rest. Sciatica with weakness and tremblings. General aggravation by long privation of sleep, vehicular disease.

Colocynthis (6, 30, 200, M)—Right sided. Aggr. in the evening, at night, by movement, by the stretching of limbs. Keeps the limbs stretched ; by contract, by cold. Amel. by rest, by hot application. Very important remedy. Sciatica with intolerable pains followed by numbness and paresis. General agar. by anger.

Dioscorea (6, 30)—Right sided. Aggr. when getting up, while walking, by movement. Amel. by rest, by slow extension (contrary to colocynthis). Cramping pain along the nerve, specially in the hip. Amel. of all symptoms by extension.

Ferrum Metallicum (6, 30)—Indifferent laterality. Aggr. by rest at night being seated. By cold, by air current. Amel. by moderate movement, by heat. Tearing pain. Pale and flushed individual, has gushes of heat, localised of the face. Anemia, chlorosis.

Gelsemium (6)—Indifferent laterality. Aggr. by rest, at the beginning of movement, at night. Chronic sciatica. Stubborn cases remedy of tremblings.

Hypericum (6)—Indifferent laterality. Aggr. by cold, humidity, mist, confined air, by touch Amel. no marked modality. Hypersensitiveness of nerves sensation of laceration, drawing pains. Burning pains with numbness. Traumatic sciatica. A remedy of traumatism of nerves. Coccygodyna. Sometime sensation as if the limbs are detached from the body.

Iris versicolor (6)—Left sided. Aggr. at night, by lying on the painful side, by cold, by touch. Amel. by walking, heat, by bending forward. Lumber neuralgia. Pain in the back, feels the need of a support. Weakness of the lumber muscles. Sometimes, numbness of the limbs. General condition depressed. General aggr. by fatigue, by sexual acts.

Kali Iodatum (6, 30)—Right sided (non-exclusive). Aggr. at night, by lying on the painful side. Amel. by movement, by walking, in open air.

syphilitic ground. Mercurial sciaticas. Pain in the posterior part of the hip with contractions and spasms of the muscles. General characteristics : Pains that forces the patient to get up at night with need for movement and cold air.

Kalmia (6)—Right sided (non-exclusive), Aggr. by bending double, by movement, by cold. General amelioration by eating. Pain from above downwards, lightning like pains. Fulgurating pains. Sensations of weakness and coldness of the lower limbs with numbness.

Lac Canimum (6)—Erratic pains passing from one side to the other. Aggr. at night, by touch, by movement. Amel. by open air. Pain in the sacral region, extending throughout a limb, disturbing sleep and rest. General aggravation during menses.

Ledum Paluster (6, 30)—Left sided (non-exclusive). Aggr. at night, by heat of the bed, by touch, by movement. Amel. by cold foot bath by applications of cold, open air and rest. Pinching pains, drawing in the whole limb, specially in the posterior face of the hip. Contraction. Joints of the feet painful, deformed, cold to touch. The affected limb is more cold than other parts of the body. Affected joints are white and not red. A good antidote of excess of wine. Rheumatic ground.

Magnesiu Phos (6)—Right sided. **Aggr.** by immobility, while lying down, by prolonged movement, by cold. Amel. by moderate movement, by heat. Pains coming and going suddenly. Fulgurating pains. Cramps, Paroxistic attacks which obliges the patient to change position, to stand up, to walk agitation. Chronic of Colocynthis. Its place is between Arsenic and Colocynthis.

Mezereum (6)—Indifferent laterality. Amel. in open air, at dawn. Burning lancinating pains with shivering. Itching syphilitic ground.

Palladium (6, 30)—Right side. **Aggr.** at night, by cold, by touch, by movement. Amel. by heat and rest. Very acute pains going from toe to the hip. Proud character, irritable, cannot support contradictions. Pain in the right ovary.

Phosphorus (6, 30)—Left sided (non-exclusive). **Aggr.** at night, lying on the painful side, by cold, morning and evening. Amel. while eating; by rest, being magnetised. General aggr. by hot drinks and mental work.

Phytolacca (6, 30)—Indifferent laterality. **Aggr.** at night, after sleep, by movement, by pressure, by humid cold. Amel. by lying down, by rest and by heat. Sudden erratic pains, as if from electric shocks, often in the external or posterior face of the hip. Chronic sciatica on a syphilitic ground. Rheumatism.

Plumbum (6, 30)—Indifferent laterality. Aggr. at night, by heat, movement, light pressure. Amel. by massage, by strong pressure. Chronic sciatica, with muscular strophy. Cramping and constrictive pains. Syphilitic ground.

Pulsatilla (6, 30)—Indifferent laterality. Aggr. by heat, confined air, immobility. Amel. by movement and open air. Erratic pains. Changing of symptoms. Veinous congestion. Mentality : timid, easily weep with amel. by consolation.

Rananculus (6)—Indifferent laterality (predominantly left sided). Aggr. in rainy weather and by storm. Morning and evening, by movement, by lying on the painful side. Amel. no clear modality. Complementary *Rhus tox.* General Aggr. by changes of weather and in humid cold.

Rhus Tox (decimals, 6, 30, 200)—Indifferent laterality. Aggr. by rest. Cannot remain immobile. Constantly changes position at night, by humidity, beginning to move, lying on the back or on the right side; by fatigue by cooling after sweat. Amel. by dry and hot weather changing of position by walk; by stretching, by hot application. Tearing pains with sensation of coldness, numbness, walking of ants. Paralytic stiffness, sensation as if the tendons are very short. Sciatica in persons being drenched in water after being hot, or who have laid down in humid place. Consequence of overwork. Rheumatic ground.

Ruta (6)—Aggr. at night, by humidity, by cold application, while lying down, by rest. Amel. by movement, by walk, by heat. Stiffness and sensitiveness of tendons. Deep seated pains, bone pains. Sensation of as if bones are broken. Rheumatic sciatica. Agitation, should walk continually.

Stillingia (6)—Left sided. Aggr. in the evening, by move-ment, by walking, by cold. Amel. in morning, in dry weather, by heat and by pressure. Violent pain from hip to toe.

Syphilitic Ground :

Tellurium (6)—Right sided. Aggr. by lying on the painful side, by the least contact, by laughing and coughing, by cold, Amel. No clear modality. Pain of the backbone, of sacrum, irradiation on sciatic nerve.

Valeriana (6)—Indifferent laterality. Aggr. by standing or in any position with the feet on the ground ; by immobility. Amel. by walking, with the limbs stretched in a horizontal position, by change of position. Acute pain along the nerve.

Veratrum Album (6, 30)—Indifferent laterality. Aggr. at night, by the heat of the bed. Amel. by walking, by ambiant heat. Cramping pains. General aggr. by cold drinks.

Viscum Album (6, 30)—Indifferent laterality. Aggr. by touch, by the least movement, by cold and by lying on the left side. Amel. by rest. Grave, stubborn case ; sensation of torsion in the muscles. Limbs heavy as lead. Hypersensitiveness to contact; prostration. Arterial hypertension, arteriosclerosis.

Zincum Metallicum (6, 30)—Indifferent laterality. Aggr. while sitting, by walk, by noise, by touch. Amelioration by moderate movement (continual movement of the feet), by menstruation, following a discharge. Sciatica with weakness and trembling. Rheumatic ground. General aggr. by wine.

C. Remedies of Secondary Importance :

We are going to enumerate briefly and in alphabetical

order the last group of medicines which are useful to know, but of less value than those which we have just studied.

Angustera (6)—Aggr. by movement. Amel. by cold application. Rigidness of limbs and lameness.

Capsicum (6)—Aggr. by movement and cold. Amel. by heat. Preferably left sided.

Carbonum sulphuratum (6)—Aggr. by movement, by walking and by night.

Coffee (6, 30)—Aggr. by emotion, by movement, by noise, at night. Amel. by rest, by pressure. Intolerance of pain. Agitation. Insomnia. Sensorial hyperesthesia.

Colchicum (decimals, 6)—Aggr. by movement, by touch, at night. Amel. by heat and by rest. Arthritic ground.

Drosera (6)—Aggr. by walk and by movement. Amel. by rest. Preferably right sided.

Dulcamara—Aggr. by humid weather; consequence of suppression of sweat, of discharge. Amel. by mild and dry climate. Rheumatic ground. Sciatica as a result of cold during humid climate.

Eupatorium purpureum (6)—Aggr. by movement. Feeling as if the bones and muscles are bruised. Feels the bed very hard. Weak legs, as if paralysed. Left sided.

Euphorbium (6)—Aggr. by movement; Amel. by rest. Great difficulty to rise from a sitting position.

Ginseng (6)—Aggr. at night and by sitting position. Sensation of deep contusion of fracture.

Hepar sulphur (6, 30)—Aggr. by movement, by walk, by the least cold. Amel. by rest and by heat. Extreme sensitiveness too cold, to the least change of weather, to air currents.

Indigo (6)—Aggr. while sitting; by rest. Amel. by movement (which is however slightly painful). Preferably right sided.

Kali Phos (6)—Aggr. by cold and by continued movement. Amel. by heat and moderate movement.

Magnesia carb (6)—Aggr. at night, by rest, by noise, by touch. By cold and at an interval of every three weeks. Amel. by movement, walking, in open air, by heat. Intolerable pains with sweats. Hyperesthesia of the skin.

Menvanthes (6)—Aggr. by walking, by rest, by going up. Amel. by strong pressure.

Mercurius (6)—Aggr. at night, while lying down, by movement. Amel. in open air, in the morning. Tearing pains along the limb. Sensation of internal heat. Skin cold. Weakness of the limb. Syphilitic and rheumatic ground.

Finally I must say a few words regarding some adjuvant methods of which the importance should not be neglected. Inspite of the rich therapeutic arsenal of Homoeopathy, homoeopaths should not forget the Thermal cures that may render good service to the patients of *Sciatiea* specially for relapsing cases.

Acupuncture and centrotherapy often, in the hands of masters, give instantaneous results. Finally in all cases of *Sciatica* gymnastic movements, active or passive are really useful where judicious treatment completely fails, or the amelioration is not satisfactory.

CHRONIC RHEUMATISM

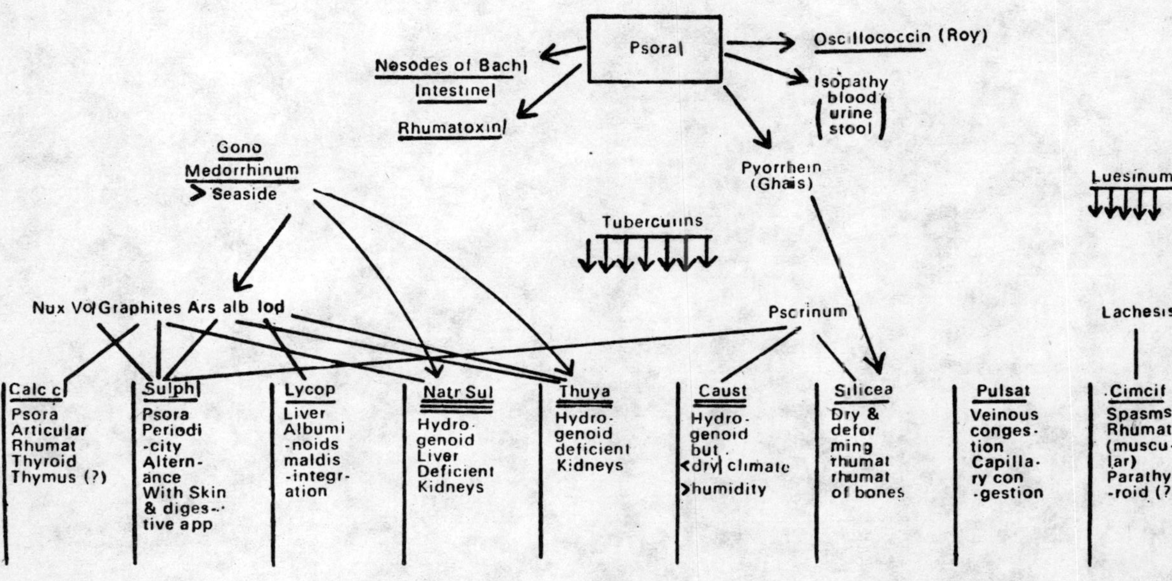

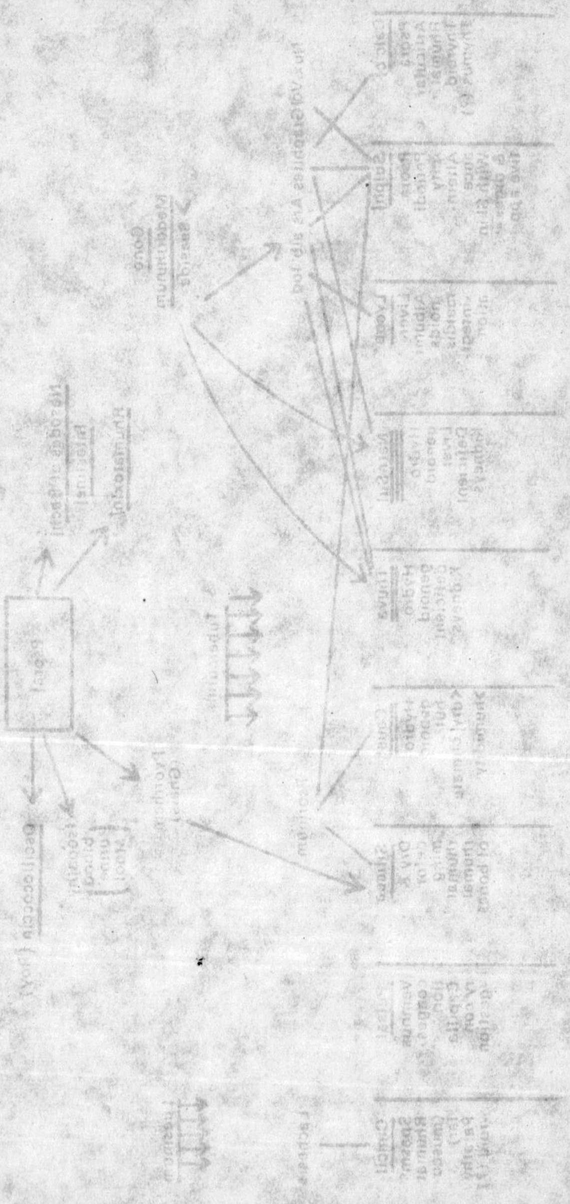